How Do I Know It's Yucky?

and other questions about the senses

by

Sharon Cromwell

Photographs by

Richard Smolinski, Jr.

Series Consultant

Dan Hogan

MOONDRAKE

First published in Great Britain by Moondrake
Halley Court, Jordan Hill, Oxford OX2 8EJ,
a division of Reed Educational & Professional Publishing Ltd

OXFORD FLORENCE PRAGUE MADRID ATHENS MELBOURNE
AUCKLAND KUALA LUMPUR SINGAPORE TOKYO IBADAN
NAIROBI KAMPALA JOHANNESBURG GABORONE
PORTSMOUTH NH (USA) CHICAGO MEXICO CITY SAO PAULO

First published 1997

01 00 99 98
10 9 8 7 6 5 4 3 2 1

ISBN 0 431 06153 X
This title is also available in hardback (ISBN 0 431 06152 1)

British Library Cataloguing in Publication Data

Cromwell, Sharon
How do I know it's yucky? – (Body wise)
1. Human anatomy – Juvenile literature 2. Human physiology – Juvenile literature 3. Body, Human – Juvenile literature
I. Title
612

Printed in Hong Kong by Wing King Tong Co. Ltd.

Contents

Some words are shown in bold, **like this**. You can find out what they mean by looking in the Glossary.

What are my senses?

You have five senses. They are are touch, taste, hearing, sight and smell.

You have touch receptors, or feelers, all over your body. You taste mostly with your tongue. You hear with your ears. You see with your eyes and you smell with your nose. Your brain plays a big part in all these things.

BODY FACT

You have the most touch receptors in your fingertips. That's why you often touch things with your fingertips.

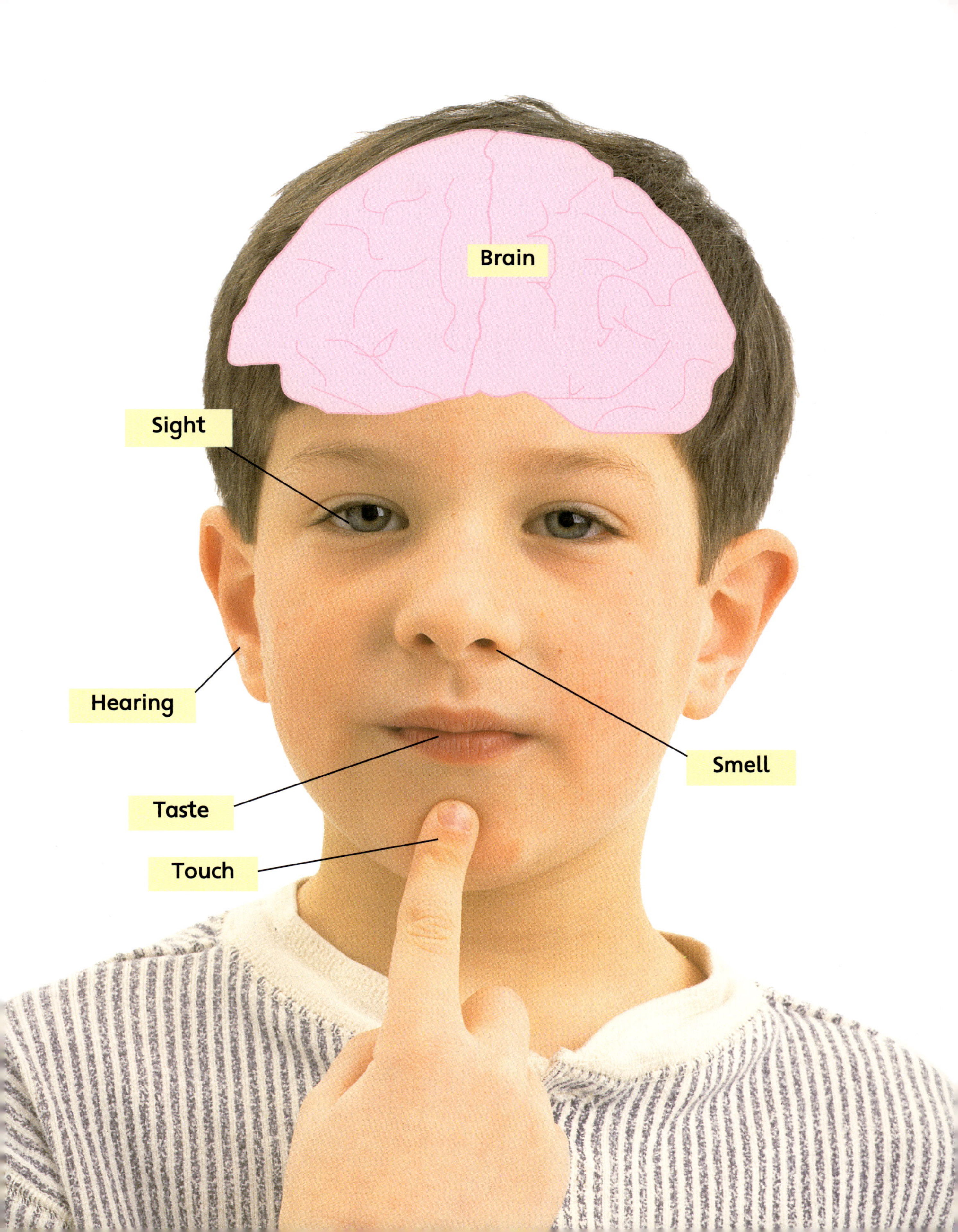
Brain
Sight
Hearing
Smell
Taste
Touch

What do my senses tell me?

Your senses tell you everything about the world around you. Your sense of touch lets you feel things. It also helps keep you safe. If you touch something very hot, you pull away from it. That keeps you from getting burned.

Your sense of hearing also helps to keep you safe. When you hear a car hooter, it is often a warning of danger. Hearing also helps you to communicate with others. Your sense of sight lets you see things all around you. This helps you move through your world safely.

BODY FACT

Your sense of taste and your sense of smell often work together. They help you decide what you want to eat and whether food is too sour!

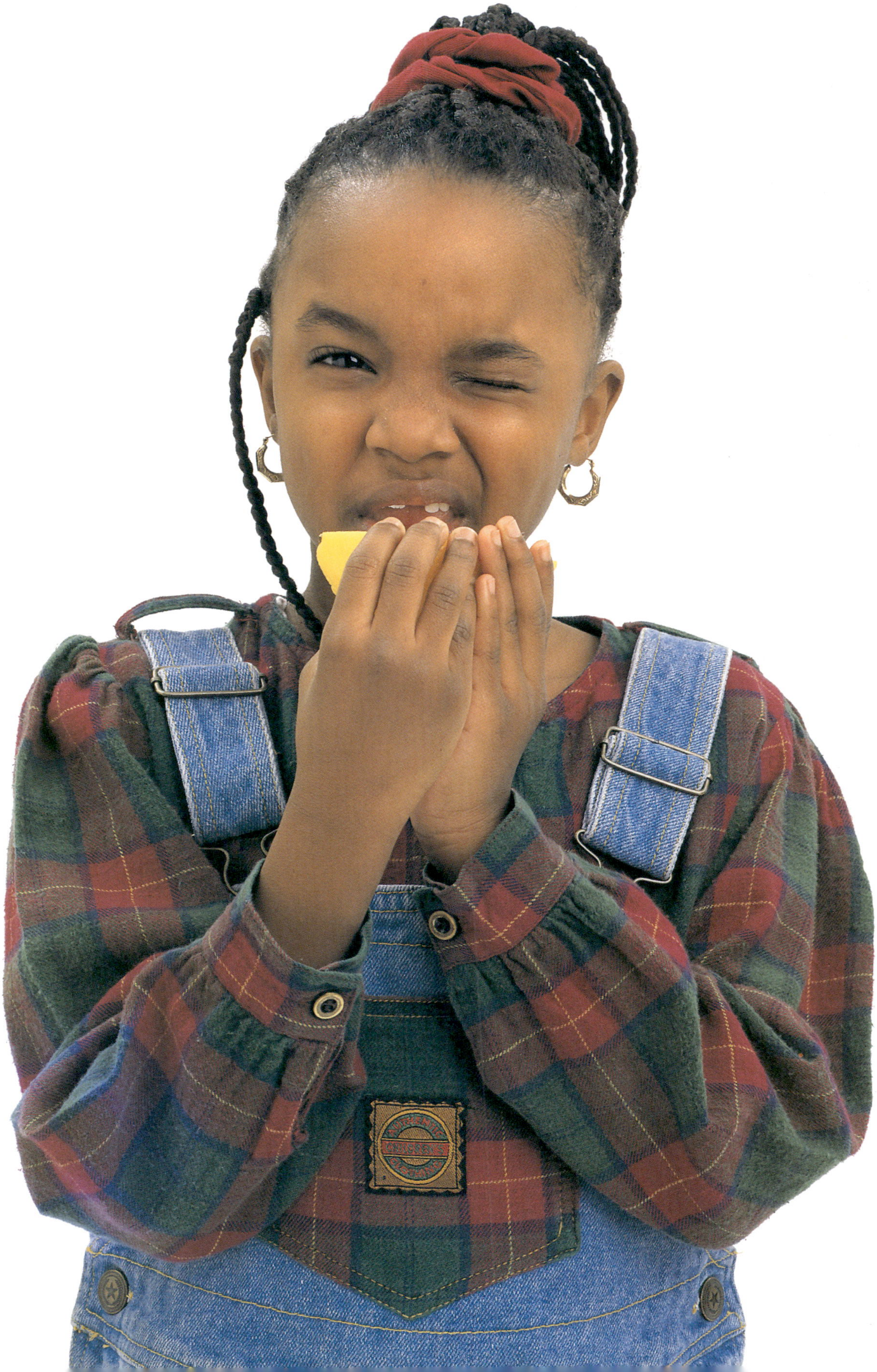

How do I feel something is itchy?

Your whole body is made up of tiny **cells**. Special cells, called receptors, are in your skin. Certain receptor cells feel itching and tickling. Let's call them feeler cells.

BODY FACT

If the part of your body swells up where you were bitten by an insect, tell a grown-up. You may be **allergic** to the insect bite.

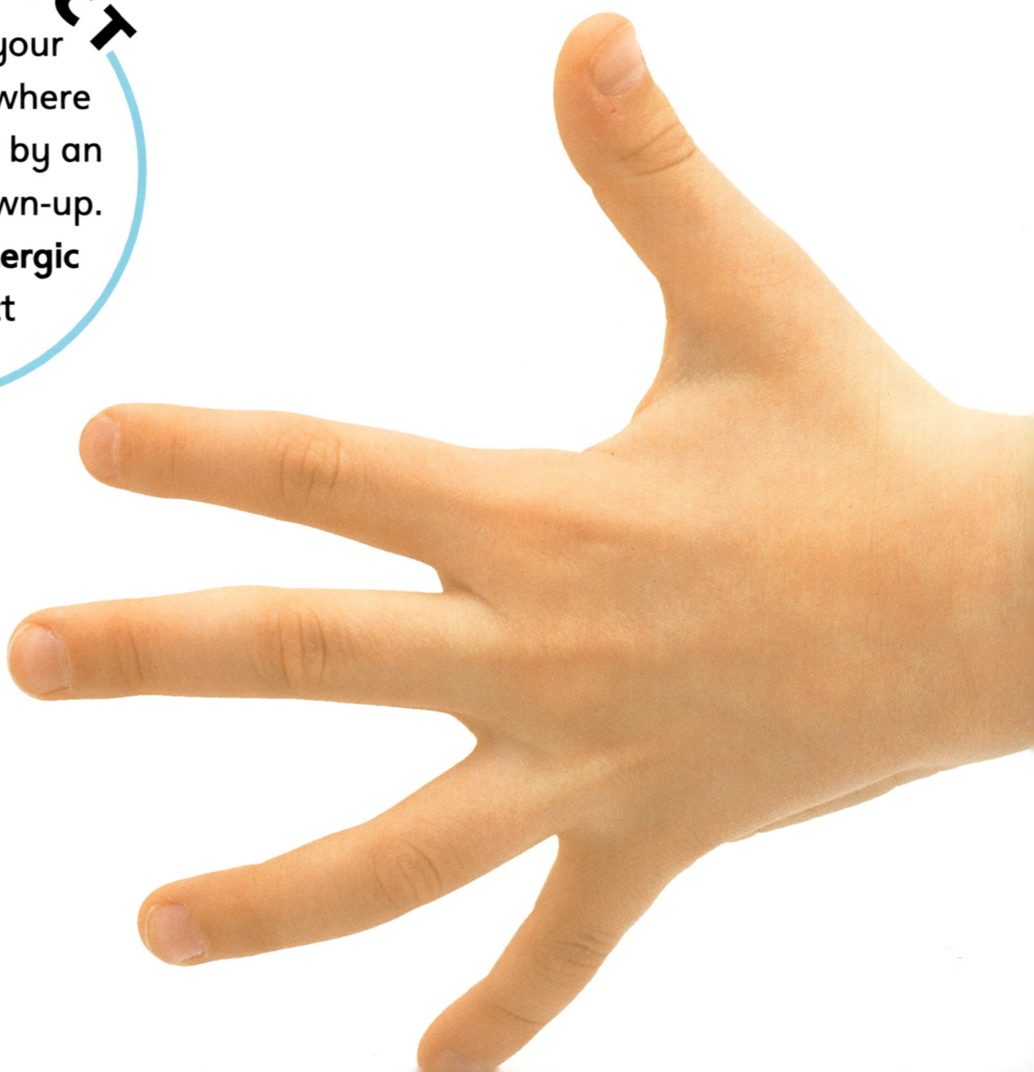

1 You have feeler cells that feel itching all over your body.

2 When your feeler cells feel an itch on your arm or some other part of your body, they send a message through your nerves to your brain.

3 Your brain sends a message to the muscles in your arm and hand.

4 Then you scratch the place that itches.

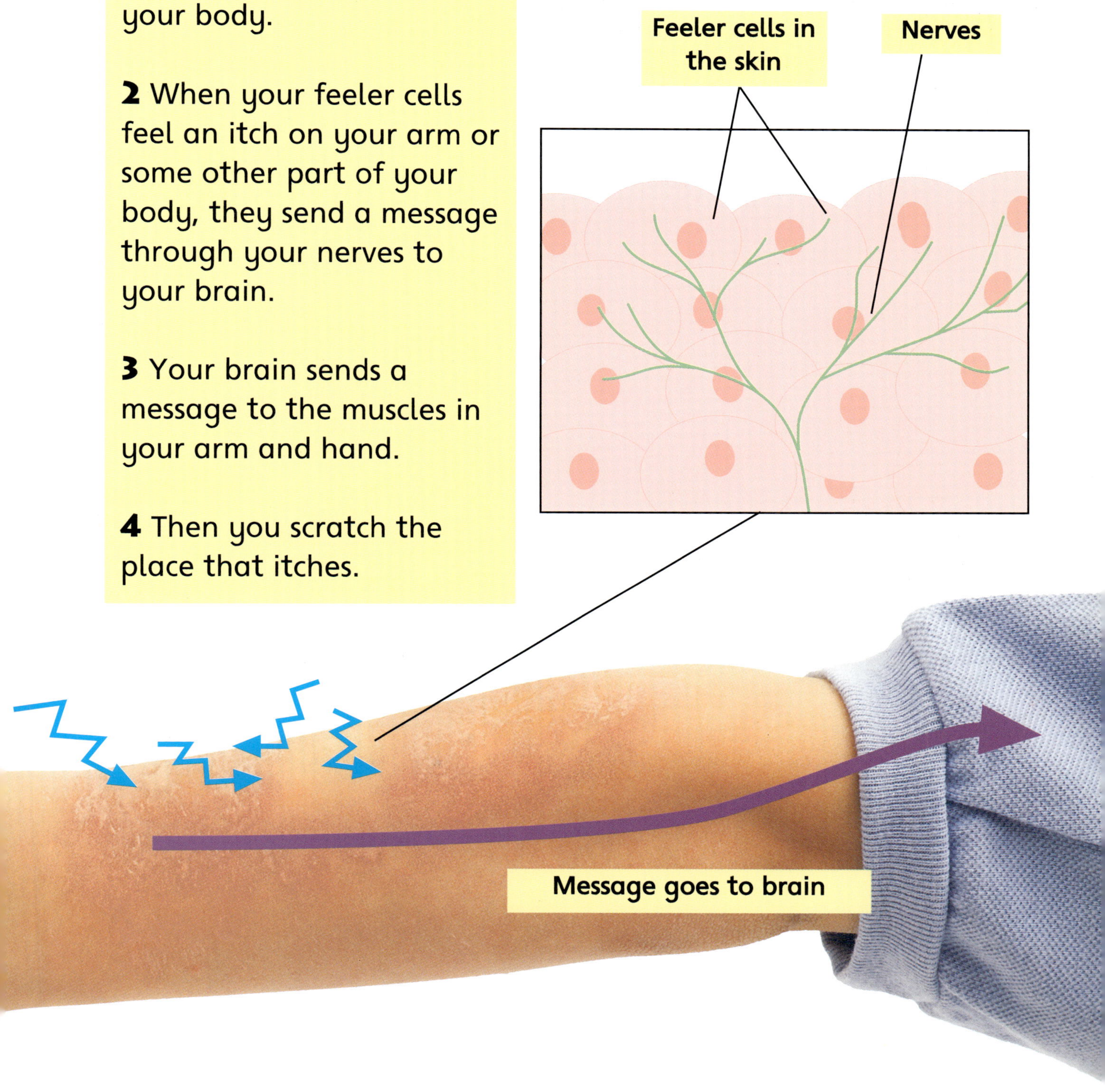

How do I know my dirty socks smell yucky?

Your nose and your brain work together so you can smell different smells and tell them apart.

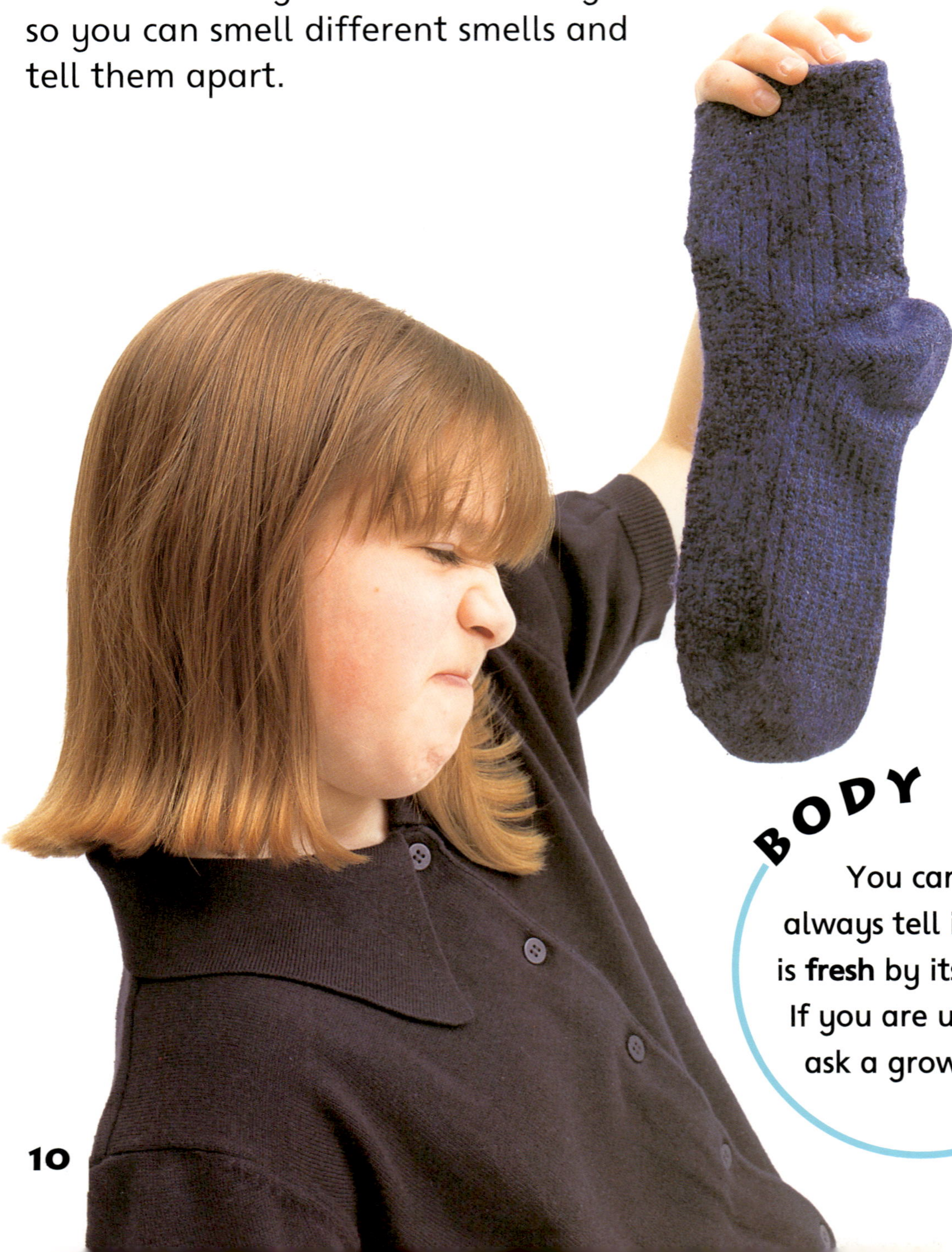

BODY FACT

You can't always tell if food is **fresh** by its smell. If you are unsure, ask a grown-up.

1 Smells are made up of tiny parts that are called molecules. They enter your nostrils.

2 Inside your nose are millions of feeler **cells** that are sensitive to smells. These cells send a message to the smell centre of the brain.

3 The smell centre of the brain identifies the smell.

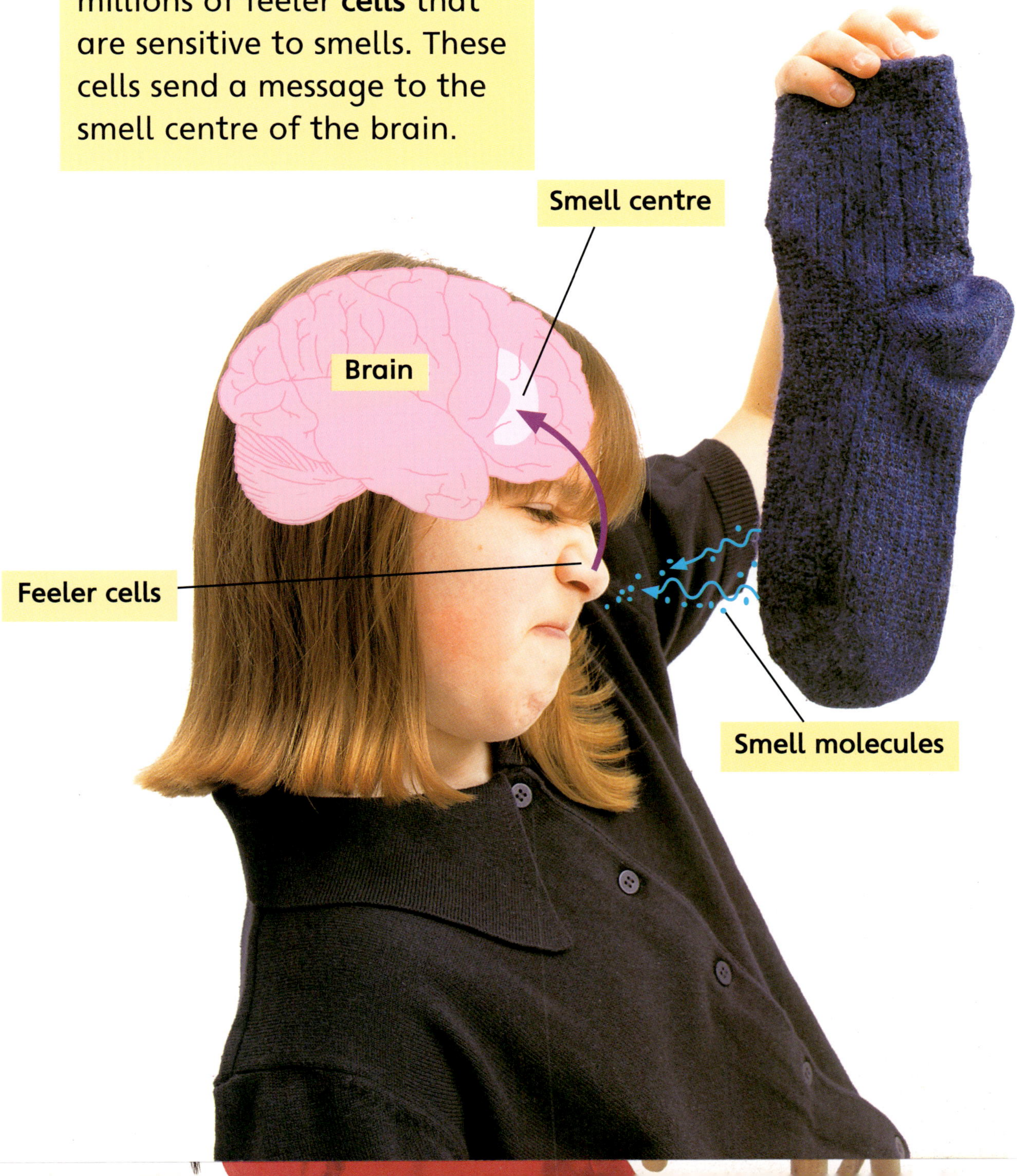

How do I taste bitter, sweet, salty and sour foods?

Tiny bumps on your tongue called taste buds let you taste.

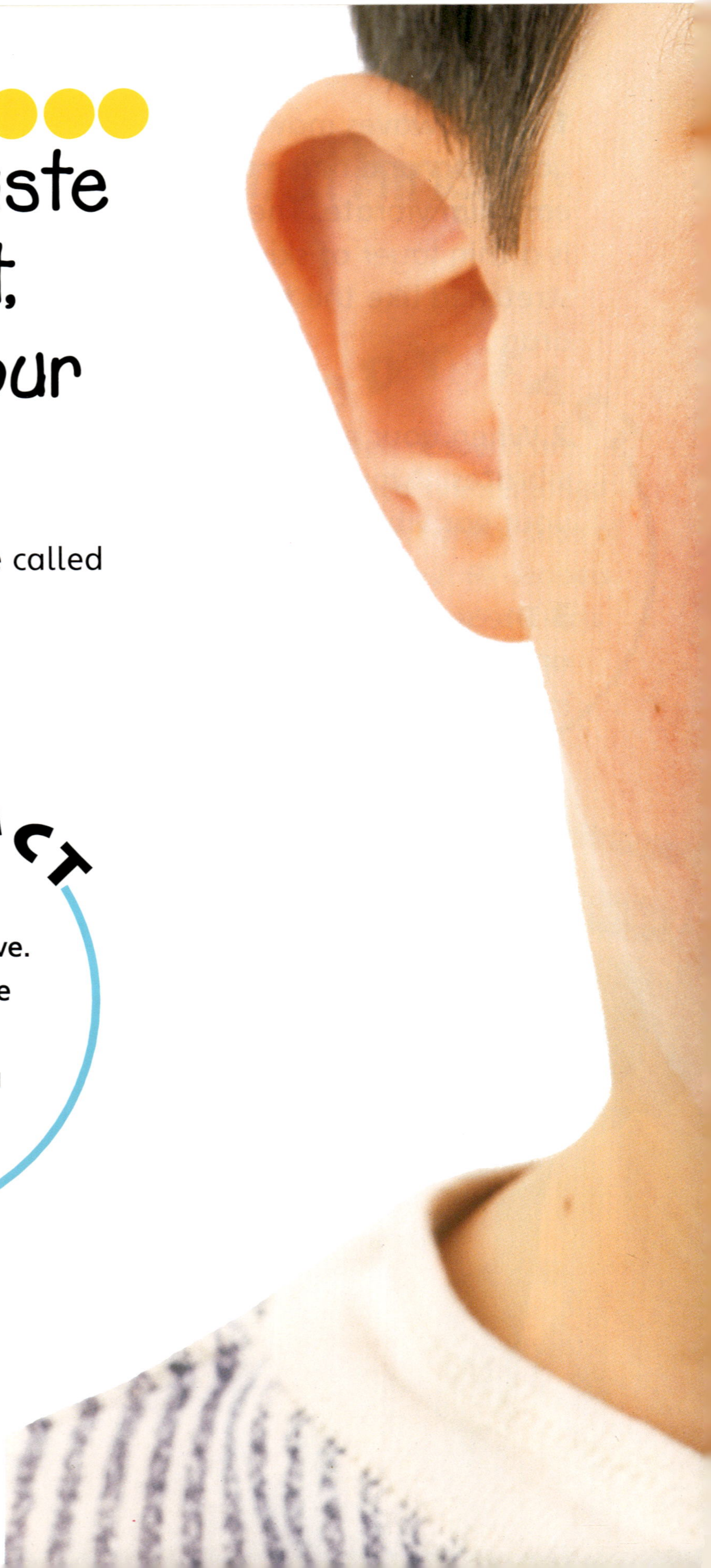

BODY FACT

Eating cold food makes your taste buds less sensitive. If you suck on an ice cube before taking some medicine, you won't notice the taste.

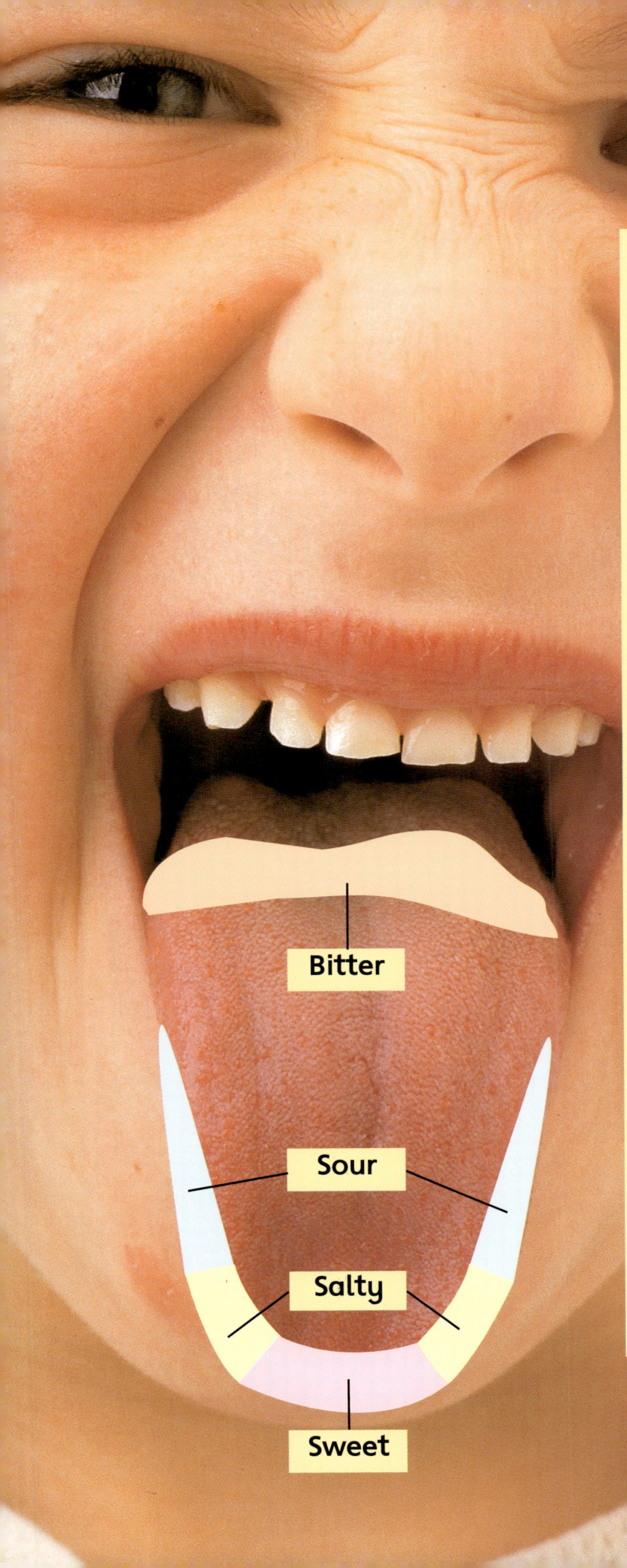

1 Taste buds are made up of feeler **cells** that take in the taste of foods.

2 You have four kinds of taste buds. These taste buds know whether something is sweet, sour, salty or bitter.

3 When you chew food your taste buds are **activated** by different foods that taste sweet, sour, salty or bitter. So if you eat something salty, like a potato crisp, the salt taste buds work.

4 The taste buds send messages to your brain that you are eating something salty.

5 Your brain then knows what you are eating.

Why can't I taste food when I have a cold?

It is hard to taste food when you have a cold because the senses of taste and smell work together.

BODY FACT

When you have a cold, try taking a hot shower to clear your nose. You will be better able to taste your food.

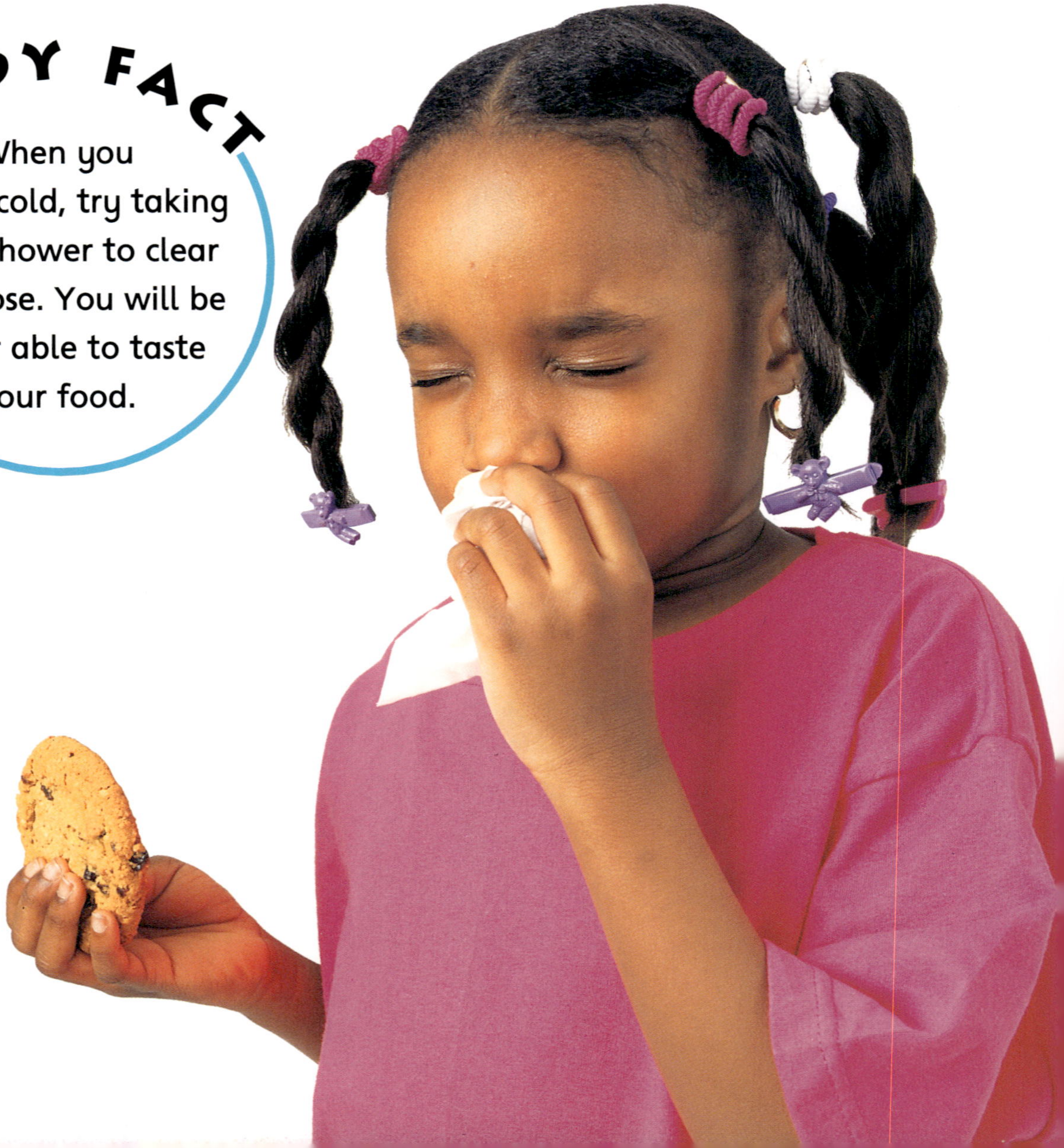

1 The stuffy nose that you often have with a cold makes it difficult to smell.

2 Your taste buds detect only four simple tastes of salty, sweet, bitter and sour. Your nose and sense of smell do much of the rest of the work of tasting!

3 The smell molecules from food give your brain much of the information it needs to identify the food.

4 When you can't smell the many **aromas** of food, you lose much of your ability to taste it.

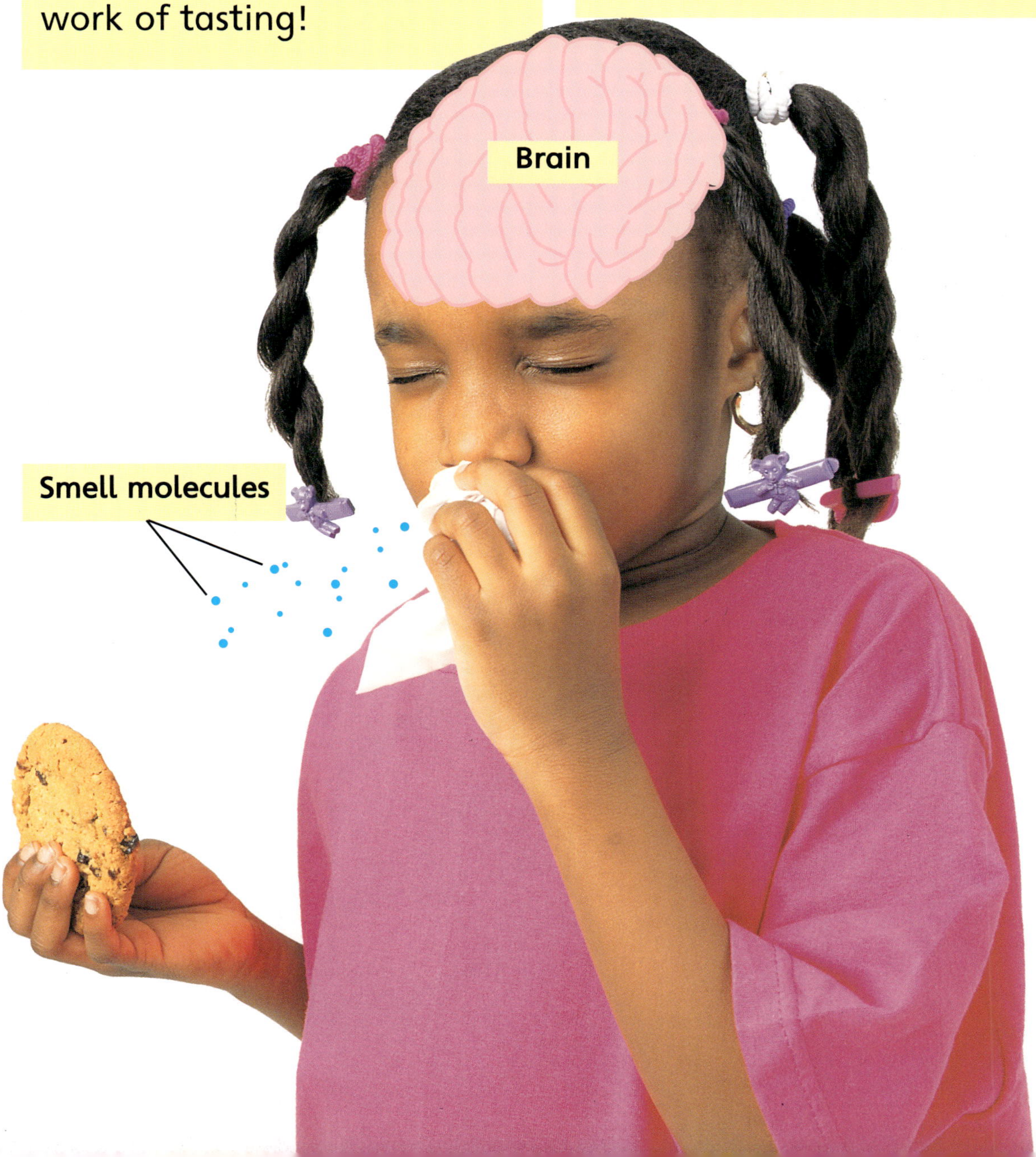

How do I know whether something is rough or smooth?

Feeler cells in your fingertips help you feel whether an object is rough or smooth.

BODY FACT

When you rub your skin against something rough many times, your skin protects itself by forming a thick outside layer called a callus.

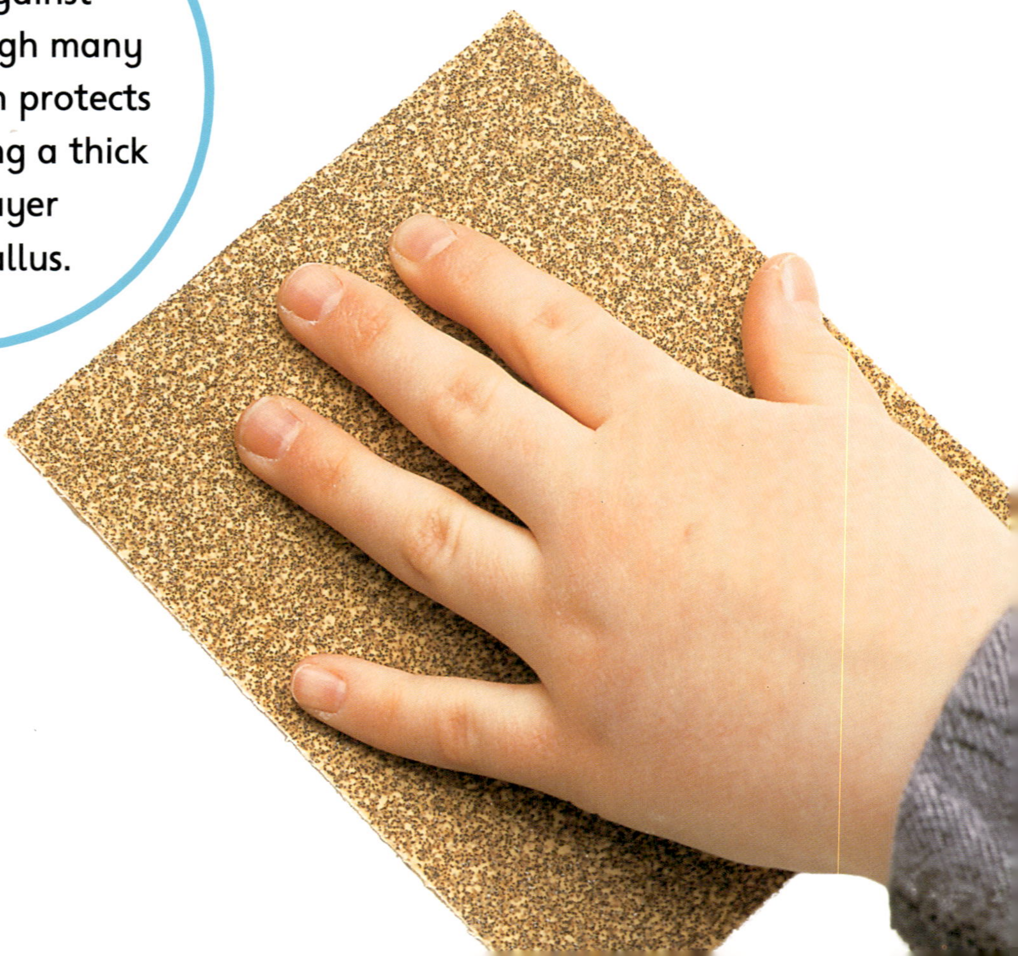

1 Feeler **cells** in your fingertips feel texture – whether something is rough or smooth. Your hand has more feeler cells than most parts of your body.

2 When you touch an object, a message about its texture goes from your feeler cells through your nerves to your brain.

3 Your brain tells you whether the object is rough or smooth.

4 If it is rough, like sandpaper, you will probably pull your hand away. If the object is soft and silky, like the fur of a pet, you may decide to stroke it.

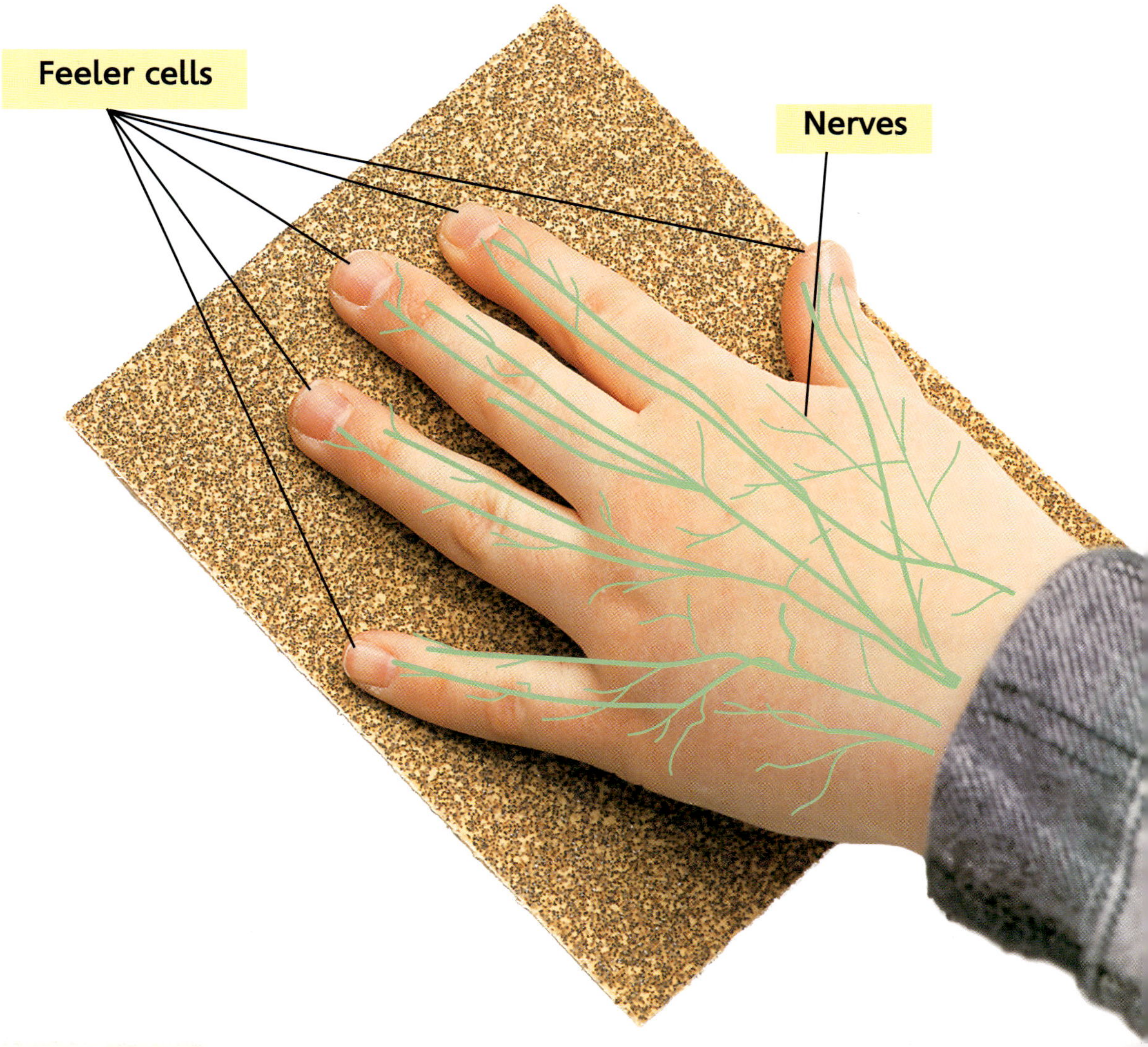

How do my eyes see colour?

Two kinds of light receptors are at the back of your eyes. One kind of light receptor takes in colour.

BODY FACT

Apricots, carrots and other orange-coloured fruits and vegetables have an important vitamin called vitamin A. It helps your eyes to see when the light is poor.

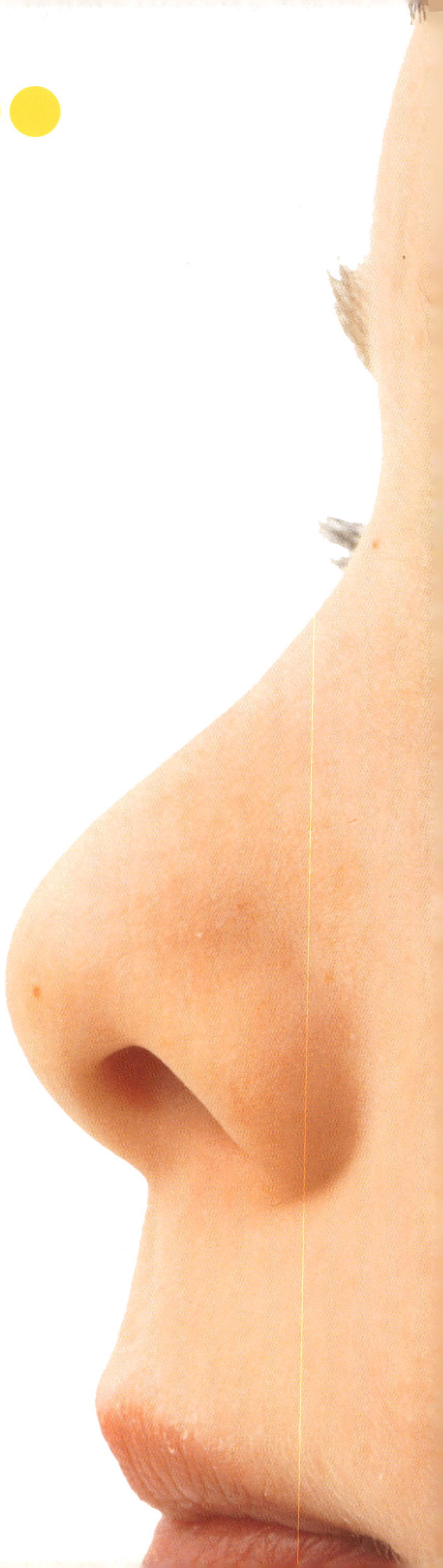

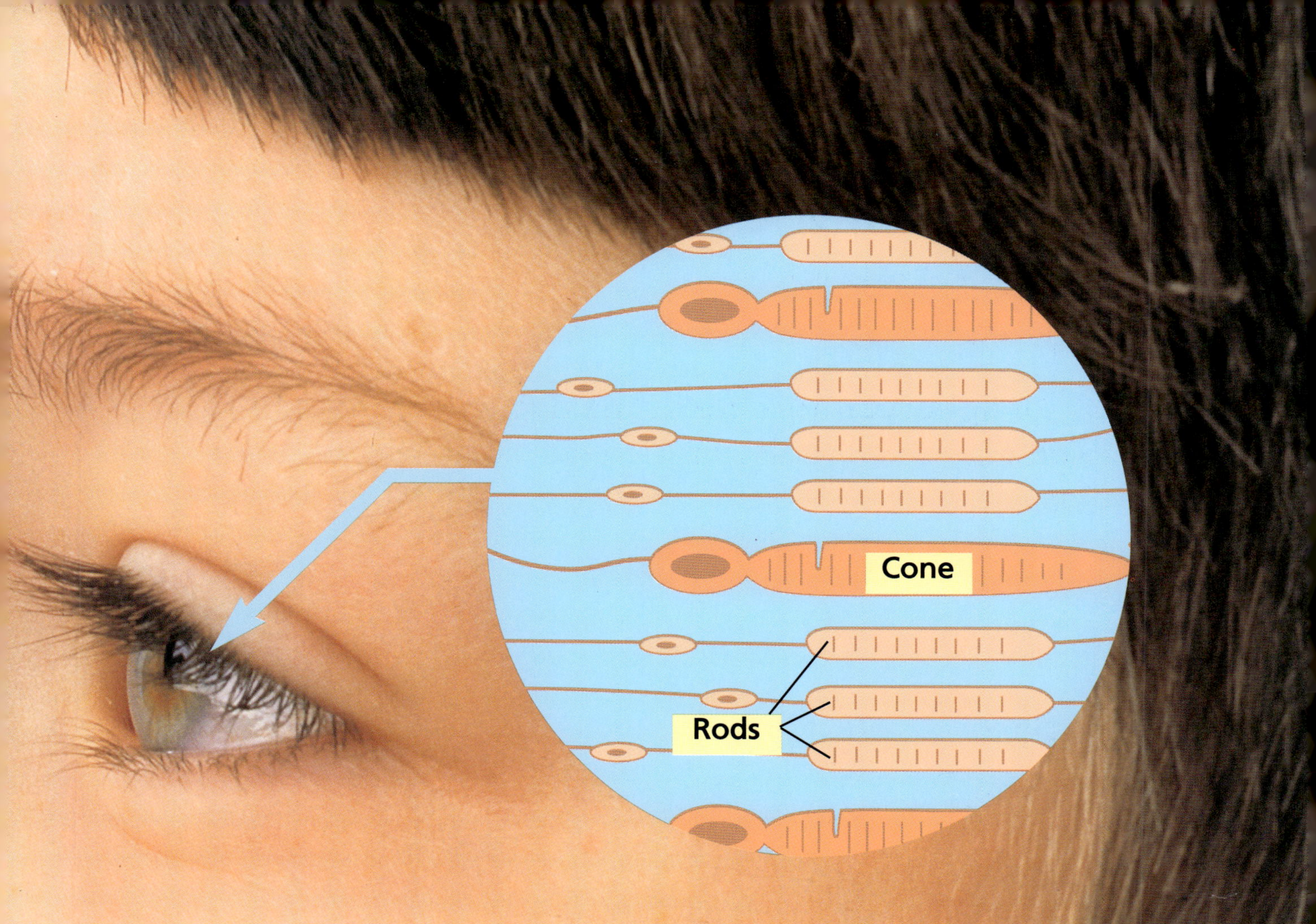

1 The two kinds of light receptors at the back of your eyes are called rods and cones. All together, the human eye has about 135 million rods and cones.

2 Rods are **cells** that are sensitive to light and dark. Three kinds of cones are receptor cells for three different colours.

3 One kind of cone receives red. Another kind receives blue. The third kind receives green.

4 Messages to the brain from the three kinds of cones combine to make all the colours you see. You can see millions of colours, all made up from those red, blue and green receiving cones.

Explore more! Your senses

1 GET TOUCHY!

WHAT YOU'LL NEED:

- water
- ice cubes
- 2 containers

THEN TRY THIS!

Pour water and some ice cubes into one container. Stir them until the water is very cold. Put some cool water in a second container. Put your hand in the ice water and leave it there as you count to 20. Take your hand out and put it into the cool water. What does the cool water feel like? Compared to ice-cold water, cool water feels warm.

2 IN GOOD TASTE!

WHAT YOU'LL NEED:

- salt
- 250ml glass of water

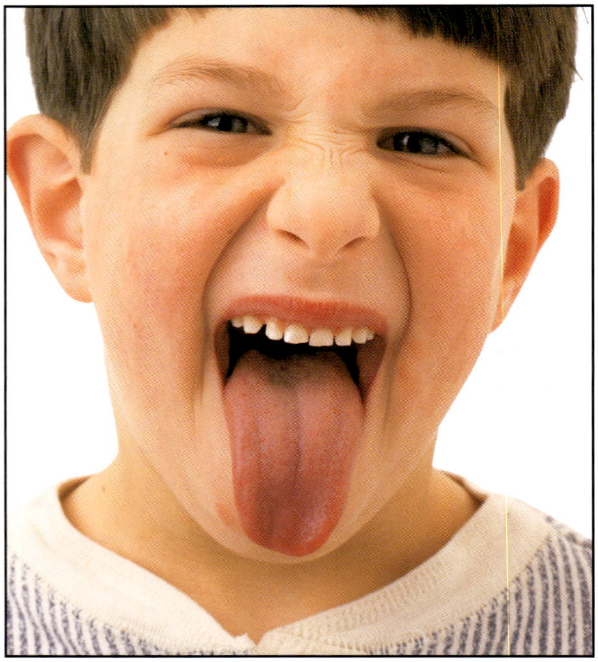

THEN TRY THIS!

Put 2 teaspoons of salt in a 250ml glass of water. Then put some salty water on the back of your tongue. Next put some salty water on the front. How did the salty water taste on the back of your tongue? How did it taste on the front? Can you tell which part of your tongue has your salt taste buds?